See YOU at the TOP

A Practical Guide to Getting off the Couch and Reaching your Fitness Goals

COACH OBASI

DEDICATION

To my brother Steve Miller who was with us for 31 years before he passed away from complications of Type 1 Diabetes. Watching him struggle to control his illness was painful and it's because of him that I began a career in health and fitness. My mission is to help people learn to use exercise and nutrition to live healthy, productive, and meaningful lives.

CONTENTS

PREFACE

When I first thought about writing this book, I was a little skeptical about it. There are already countless fitness books out there written by people who have more experience and expertise than I do. I wanted to put together a simple guide to help people sort through all the confusing information and begin the journey to good health. I've worked as a personal trainer and nutrition coach for about 7 years at a commercial gym in St. Louis, Missouri. I've had the opportunity to train, advise, and help hundreds of people. I've learned a thing or two about working out, healthy eating, why some people reach their goals, and why others don't.

Most of the people I've worked with don't know it, *but I'm a borderline diabetic.* That means my blood sugar levels are higher than normal, but not high enough to have full diabetes. At this point, I don't take medication of any kind. I monitor my glucose levels, work out consistently, and watch my carb intake very closely. I have a family history of diabetes and high blood pressure, so I don't take any of this lightly. I want to be as healthy as I can, for as long as I can. If you're reading this and are dealing with an illness, hopefully you feel the same way.

I never imagined working as a fitness professional. I really fell into it. Before moving to St. Louis in 2011, I lived in New Jersey and worked for years as an elementary school teacher. I had a few other jobs, but nothing remotely related to fitness. Throughout the years, I played basketball, jogged, and did a ton of push-ups, but I never went to the gym consistently. Like many people, I'd exercise for a few months, and then drop off, but I'd always start up again out of the fear of gaining weight. The transition from educator to personal trainer was an easy one for me because the skill set is *very* similar. You must be an effective communicator, with an emphasis on being a good *listener*. You must motivate and inspire clients (students) to do things they don't think they can do. I often tell people that I'm still a teacher, but instead of teaching children how to read and do math, I'm teaching adults about exercise and nutrition. To be successful with either group, you need passion and commitment.

Whether you're new to fitness, or you've been working out for a while, I want you to succeed. I want you to lose the weight. I want you to get stronger and increase your endurance. I want you to feel better, look better, and be better. I want you to be more confident and knowledgeable about your body and your health. If you're looking for practical exercise and nutrition information that (if utilized) will help you reach your goals, this book is for you!

INTRODUCTION

After a long day at work, one of my clients came in for her regular training session. She warmed up on the treadmill and did a few stretches. As we were getting ready to do a set of deadlifts, she turned to me with this look on her face and said, "Obasi I don't feel like working out, but I know I have to." I'd heard those words in the gym many times before, but for some reason on that day it really hit me. I thought to myself, "That's it!" Most people don't really like working out, as a matter of fact, some of them hate it. They do it because they're tired of being overweight. They're tired of their clothes fitting too tight. They're tired of getting out of breath after climbing a flight of stairs. They're tired of not being able to keep up with their kids or grandchildren. They're tired of taking medication. Yes, there are some people who love lifting weights and doing cardio, but most people work out because they want results, even if they don't enjoy the process. At the end of the day, we work out because deep down we know *we have to*!

Let's be honest. If there was a pill we could take to lose weight for good, without doing any exercise, most people would buy it. If there was some magical way we could get the body we want without putting in the work, we'd jump at the opportunity. But, we all know it doesn't work that way. If you want results you're going to have to make some sacrifices. You'll have to put in the work and make some lifestyle changes. You're going to have to change your approach toward eating. Yes, it's going to be challenging and even frustrating at times. Believe me when I say, "Your health is worth the struggle."

People from all over the world have made the decision to lead healthier lives by exercising regularly and changing their eating habits. So, the good news is you're not alone. There are plenty of resources to help you navigate the road to fitness. Be careful though, because the road that leads to fitness and health won't be a smooth one. It will get bumpy at times and will be full of unexpected obstacles. Don't get discouraged, because if you keep going, you can make it.

One of the challenges you'll face is sorting through the avalanche of information available online. There are some good websites out there with reliable exercise and nutrition information, but we all know you can't believe everything you read on the Internet. So, make sure you get information from a credible source. There are many trainers and coaches who have dedicated their lives to helping others change their behavior and build new bodies. Do yourself a favor. Find a good one and don't be afraid to make an investment in yourself. You can pay a trainer or coach to help you get in shape, or you can pay a doctor or surgeon to treat a lifestyle-related illness. Either way, you are going to pay!

A client I've worked with off and on over the years, was given three months by her doctor to lose weight and get her blood pressure under control. She called me, and we started discussing concerns she had about her health. We talked about hypertension and diabetes, and how these are diseases we can do something about. In other words, making lifestyle changes can sometimes reverse these conditions, or reduce the need for medication. We also talked about how people abuse themselves for years with unhealthy food and lack of exercise, and how unfair it is to expect our spouses, siblings, or children to step in and take care of us when we get sick. Anyone, of course, can be diagnosed with a debilitating disease, no matter how much they exercise and eat right. But taking better care of yourself can decrease the odds of becoming a burden to your family and friends.

The road to health and fitness is a journey, and you won't get there overnight. You will be faced with all kinds of challenges along the way. Life won't stop because you decide it is time to get in shape. We still work, go to school, take care of our families, etc. Unfortunately, friends and family members might not be as supportive as you expect. You might even have to remove some folks from your immediate circle. The journey will be hard enough without having negative people in your life and in your space.

See, here's the thing! Sometimes the people around us have some of the same struggles as we do. If you're dealing with weight issues, some of your friends may be in the same boat. Your decision to change might make them uncomfortable and force them to look at themselves. If they are not ready to do that, they may end up trying to sabotage your efforts. The main obstacle, however, is you! You must conquer the space between your ears by controlling negative self-talk and working toward eliminating the doubt you have about your ability to make change. *You* will be the greatest challenge, as you move toward physical and mental health. Once you understand that success is only a matter of time and effort, you'll be willing to do whatever it takes to reach your goals. Those who reach their goals are the ones who don't quit. They might feel like giving up from time to time, but they don't give in to the temporary emotion that makes us want to fall back into our comfort zones when things get tough. It's time for you to be uncomfortable, because that's how you're going to get results.

CHAPTER 1

GOAL *Setting is the* SECRET *Sauce*

You've made the decision to get started and you're finally going to do it. You're finally going to lose the weight and work on improving your health. Congratulations on taking the first step! Before you do anything, I want you to sit down and establish some goals. What do you want to look like? What do you want to be able to do? How do you want to feel? In addition to setting clear goals (the what), spend some time thinking about what will motivate or drive you to accomplish them (the why). Why do you want to lose weight? Why do you want to get stronger? Why do you want more endurance? This is a process you can't afford to skip because there will be days when you don't feel like working out or going to the gym. There will be days when you really crave pizza, or you want that large soda or iced tea. There will be times when you just want to hang out with your friends and eat what you want. It's ok. We all feel that way at times.

Your motivation will help keep you focused and help you get back on track when you stray off course. Maybe you're getting married in a year and want to lose weight to fit into that special dress. Maybe you're going on vacation and you need to drop some pounds to wear that new bathing suit. Your job might require you to do heavy lifting, and you need to strengthen your legs and back. Running a 10K or half-marathon might be on your bucket list, or your doctor told you that you need to lose weight for health reasons. Whatever your motivation is, you'll need to remind yourself of it often, especially when things get tough, and believe me *they will*.

The danger in proceeding without specific goals, is that you run the risk of wasting valuable time and achieving minimum results. Inconsistency develops when there's no plan. It's like trying to sail a ship from one location to another without a compass or navigation system. *You probably won't make it to your destination!* This situation is frustrating, but avoidable, if you take the time to set clear goals in the beginning. Don't *wing it* through your workouts and nutrition. Develop a plan and be willing to follow through with it.

There are a couple of things to consider regarding goal setting. First, it's not really a goal unless you write it down. Only a small percentage of the population have written goals, so this step alone will put you in a select group of people who are committed to success. Second, whether written out by hand, or typed on your laptop or phone, I want you to read your goals every day. Our focus here is health and fitness, but you should create goals for all areas of your life. You might be thinking, "Why do I need to read my goals every day?" Because you want them to seep into your subconscious mind and stay there. You want them to be part of your daily internal dialogue. You want to develop a constant awareness of your goals and your journey. If you never read them, it's impossible for this process to happen.

You may have heard the phrase SMART goals. This isn't a new concept, but I think this is a solid approach to goal setting. The **S** means set goals that are SPECIFIC. It's not enough to say you want to lose weight or build muscle. How much weight do you want to lose? How much muscle do you want to gain? How far do you want to run? A mile? A 5k? A marathon? Do you want to lower your body fat percentage? Do you want a leaner mid-section? Think specifically about what you really want to accomplish and set your goals accordingly.

The **M** stands for MEASURABLE. Weight loss is something you can easily measure over time simply by stepping on a scale once a week. Strength is another goal that can be measured. If you can only do 1 or 2 pull ups in January, but 6 months later you're able to do 10 or 15, we know you got stronger. If you like running, we can measure your improvement in speed or distance over time. If it's a goal that can't be measured, how will you know if you're moving in the right direction?

Let's get to **A**. Your goals should be ATTAINABLE or realistic. I could set a goal to break the world record in the 100-meter dash, but how attainable is that? I ran track way back in junior high, but no matter how much I train, how well I eat, or how much rest I get, there's no chance of breaking Usain Bolt's world record. Should goals make you stretch or step outside your comfort zone? Absolutely! Losing 60 pounds is an attainable goal because many people have done it. Will the pursuit of this goal make you uncomfortable at times? Yes, it will. Maybe you want to squat 2x your body weight. Is this an attainable goal? Yes. Will it be a major struggle for some people? There's no doubt about it, but it's still reachable. The point is, set goals that are attainable, but that also make you work to reach them.

R is for RELEVANT. How important are your goals? Are they worth your time and effort? Will they still be important in 5 or 10 years? For example, lowering your blood pressure will have a long-term impact on your life and your health. Losing weight will take pressure off your knees which may help you avoid injury or knee replacement surgery. These are goals that can greatly improve the quality of your life for years to come. So, when you set your goals make sure they're relevant to you, your family, your lifestyle, and your values.

The last step is **T**. It's my belief that all goals should have a TIMETABLE attached to them. If you don't set a deadline, it's like giving yourself an excuse to fail or give up. If you tell me you want to lose 30 pounds, I'm going to ask you, "By what date do you want to lose it?" Setting a date will help hold you accountable and it ties back into goals being measurable. If your goal is to lose 30 in six months and you've only lost 10 by the 5th month, it's going to be tough. Unfortunately, I know people who've been trying to lose the same 25 to 30 pounds for years. They may have set a goal, but because they never established a timetable, there was no accountability. It's easy to let yourself off the hook when you don't have anyone to answer to. Don't let this happen to you.

Earlier I talked about establishing your motivation. This is the why *behind* the what. It's important to spend time thinking about this. If your motivation isn't strong enough there's a good chance that you'll give up before you reach your goals. Your motivation doesn't have to be anything huge, but it should keep you going when you feel like quitting. It should also be something you remind yourself of constantly. Let's say there's a pair of jeans you haven't worn in years and you really want to get back into them. Hang them up in your room or closet so that every time you get dressed, you can see them. This will serve as a powerful reminder of why you're working hard in the gym and changing your eating habits.

After writing down your goals, I recommend posting them around the house, so that they're visible. The bathroom mirror and the refrigerator are ideal places because we walk past them often. We start our day in the bathroom, and eventually make it to the kitchen. Why is it important to post your goals? Because you want to saturate your sub-consciousness with them. You want constant reminders of the new body and new life you're working to create. You want to wake up thinking about them and go to sleep with the same thoughts. Also, don't be afraid to share your goals with supportive friends and family. They can help hold you accountable when you start slipping. Consequently, the more you talk about your goals, the better chance you have of succeeding. Goal setting, along with taking direct action, allows you to get what you want.

Surround yourself with like-minded people who can serve as a support system as you move forward. It's also important to figure out who wants you to succeed, and who doesn't. The next statement might shock you. *Not all your friends and family members want you to be successful.* As a matter of fact, there are people in your life who may try to sabotage your efforts to lose weight. It's sad, but true. Unfortunately, it may be someone close to you who throws up roadblocks, hoping that you'll fail. It may be your spouse or significant other. It might be a sibling, parent, or a close friend. You cannot allow *anyone* to stand in the way of what you need to do. In the case of a spouse or mate, it's important to sit down and let them know what you're doing, and why it's important to you. You also want to let them know how they can support you. For example, if your mate does the grocery shopping, ask them to buy foods that support the lifestyle changes you're making. Even better, go grocery shopping together so they understand which foods you need.

Family members are one thing, but when it comes to friends who aren't supportive, you may have to remove them from your circle. You don't need negative energy from people at a time when you're working to make your life better. Negative energy creates unnecessary stress, and your goal is to eliminate as much of it as possible. Added stress can potentially make it harder to lose weight. Someone once told me, *"Not everyone can sit on your front row!"* You want to reserve those seats for the most positive people you know, because they'll be your biggest cheerleaders. They're the ones who will, actively and enthusiastically, do what they can to support you.

Don't misunderstand. I'm not saying that you need to cut people completely out of your life, but you may have to stay away from them while you focus your attention on your goals and your health. You can choose to resume the relationships later if you want, but for now you need to surround yourself with positive, uplifting, and goal-oriented people.

CHAPTER 2

*Can't **DRINK** From a **FIRE** Hose*

It's hard to turn on the TV or radio, without being bombarded with all kinds of commercials and ads about the hottest exercise program, or the latest miracle supplement. When you add the Internet and social media to the mix, you have a confusing, and often overwhelming, flood of information that can frustrate fitness newbies and veterans alike. Fitness is a multi-billion-dollar industry, and while most coaches and trainers do their best to teach people good exercise and nutrition habits, some companies are out to make a quick buck by selling gadgets and gimmicks you don't need. They prey on your desire to lose weight quickly, and they often make baseless claims with no real science to back them up. Please don't fall for these "lose it quick" schemes. There's no substitute for hard work and healthy eating. If you're looking for shortcuts, you're going to be disappointed and waste precious time. Making lasting change is tough, and if someone is trying to sell you something to make things easier, you should be very skeptical. I would advise you to do your own research and listen to your own common sense.

As you begin your journey, it's important to understand that you don't have to be a gym rat to reach your goals. Gym rats are people who work out almost every day, often for hours at a time. Every time you look up they're in the gym. I don't have anything against people who are extremely focused, but it's hard to maintain a balanced life, and give your body the rest it needs, if you're working out all the time.

My advice is to start with 3 days a week and just work on being consistent with that. It's fine to add a day or two down the road, but you should start with a schedule you can manage and go from there. You don't want to neglect your other responsibilities by spending all your free time working out. You can manage your career, be attentive to your significant other, spend time with your children, and get in phenomenal shape at the same time! It's about managing your time effectively, so that you can balance what's important to you away from the gym and have time to focus on your fitness goals when you're there.

So, here's the secret to experiencing new levels of health and energy. Are you ready? Here it is. *To get into the best shape of your life you have to start*! That's it. Start where you are, with what you can do, and focus on being consistent. There's a term we use to describe someone who is really out of shape. It's called *deconditioned*. People with this status have very little strength and endurance, and they've usually been inactive for a long time. If this describes you, I recommend starting slowly. Walking around your neighborhood may be a big challenge. That's ok. Walk as far as you can. Riding a stationary bike may be tough. No problem. Ride as long as you can. Doing a push-up might be out of the question. Start with a modified version. The point is not to worry about what you can't do. Start where you are, and you'll get stronger and healthier over time, if you don't quit!

Whether you prefer lifting weights, running, biking, swimming, or taking classes, the point is to get moving by doing something you like. I can't emphasis this enough. If you're doing something you enjoy, you're more likely to stick with an exercise program. Personally, I like weight training because it has benefits you won't get from other activities. But it's better to start doing something, instead of continuing to do nothing. Your goals, and working with a fitness professional, will help determine which activities are best for you.

Millions of people are losing weight and changing their lives, so there's no reason to think you can't do the same! There are thousands of coaches, trainers, nutritionists, and other health professionals, willing to work with you and help you achieve your goals. You may even have family members and friends who've already committed to some of the lifestyle changes you seek. Sit down and talk to them to find out what they're doing. If you join a gym, you'll have no problem meeting people just like you, who have some of the same goals, and have faced some of the same challenges.

If you're new to this, understand that *you can't make up for years of inactivity in a few workouts.* It's going to take time, and your goal is to build your body slowly. I've watched far too many people pound themselves into the ground during their first couple of months. Trying to do too much too fast can get you injured, and then you'll lose momentum. One of the main reasons people stop going to the gym is because they get hurt, and once that happens, the old habits and patterns start to creep back. Now, I'm not saying you won't have to work hard to reach your goals. There's no doubt about that. Nothing will come easy, but give your body time to adjust to the new stress you're placing on it. Decrease the chance of getting injured by keeping things simple. When you start getting stronger you'll be able to do more, but there's no need to rush it. Always remind yourself of why you started in the first place, and what you want to accomplish in the long run. It's not about reaching your goals as fast as you can. It's about doing it in a way that you can maintain over the long term.

Every now and then, I'll see someone doing something they probably saw in their social media feed or saw someone doing in the gym. Sometimes these exercises are very risky, and while they may get attention, a beginner probably shouldn't try them. If you decide to add a more advanced movement to your routine, determine if the risk is worth the benefit you'll gain from it. What are you trying to accomplish? What muscles are you trying to work or develop? Is there a safer or more effective way to get the same result? These are some of the questions you should think about before doing *any* exercise.

It's important to master the basic movements that will ultimately help you build muscle and develop strength. When you're doing resistance training, focus on compound movements like squats, deadlifts, rows, and presses. Sure, there are other movements you'll want to do, but these are the ones that will help you build a solid foundation. They won't necessarily get folks looking (at least until you get some heavier weight on the bar), but they will get you impressive results in the long run.

You've set some goals, established your motivation, done a little research, and thought about how you want to work out. Now it's time to find a good gym. Hopefully, you can find one that's close to where you live or work. You might be thinking, "I have a bunch of equipment at home, why do I need to join a gym?" There's nothing wrong with working out at home from time to time, but I think it's a mistake to make your home the first option. Joining a gym, for just a few dollars a month, gives you a few important benefits. You have access to a wide range of weight lifting and cardio equipment, which will allow you to vary your workouts, when necessary. You'll get support from other people just like you, who in many cases, have goals like yours. Also, you'll be in a place where you can work out without distractions.

Your gym family can be a tremendous support system, especially if you're not getting it from family members and friends. There's something powerful about surrounding yourself with people who are working to get healthy and feel better about themselves. You'll feed off their energy, and they'll pick you up when you're feeling discouraged about your progress, or feel your commitment slipping. Since gym time is your time, you can zone out for an hour or two, and focus solely on yourself. Just make sure you don't socialize too much. If you want to chat with someone *after* you finish working out, that's fine. But don't allow anyone to distract you from taking care of business. Put your headphones on and go to work!

Are you hesitant to join a gym because you feel self-conscious about your weight or how you look? I understand how you feel, and it's normal to feel that way. What I've found is that most people go about their own business and pay little attention to what others are doing. Most gyms have people of all shapes and sizes, so don't let fear or anxiety stop you. There's a young guy who works out in my gym who has a prosthetic leg. He could worry about people staring at him, but he doesn't. He goes about his business and works out as hard as anyone else. There are a couple of women who are visually impaired, and I know a few people who get around using walkers. Several folks are morbidly obese, and it would be easy for them to make excuses. They show up because they have goals like everyone else, and they do what they can. Making excuses won't get the weight off! Your health and your life are more important than worrying about how you think others might react to you.

The next thing you want to do is find a certified trainer or coach you feel comfortable with and who knows how to help you reach your goals. I can't emphasize this point enough. Working in a gym over the last 7 years, I've watched people come in with uncertified trainers. Lots of people have good intentions and know their way around the gym, but that doesn't mean you should allow them to train you. A good trainer needs to be able to do more than give you a tough workout. Anyone can make you sweat and get you breathing hard, but a good trainer understands how to progress you through workouts without causing unnecessary stress on your body. A good trainer understands how to modify movements and adapt workouts to match your fitness level. A good trainer knows how to structure a workout that addresses your strength and endurance needs. A good trainer understands how to adjust your program, when you're not getting the results you want. A good trainer is knowledgeable about nutrition and can help you develop better eating habits. A good trainer is an excellent communicator who also knows how to listen to your concerns and hold you accountable for the goals you set.

Are there knowledgeable people out there without certifications? Yes, there are. Are there people without certifications who have helped others lose weight? There are, but you might want to proceed with caution. There are people without medical degrees who are very knowledgeable about how the body works, but you wouldn't go to them if you got sick and needed medical attention. There are unlicensed people who do electrical and plumbing work, but I'm not sure you would you hire them to do major work on your house. There are tons of shade tree mechanics who work on cars all the time, but I wouldn't recommend letting them do extensive engine work on your car or truck? Here's my point. When you make the decision to improve your health and change your body, you'll need to invest in yourself. It's a big decision, so don't take shortcuts by hiring someone just to save a few dollars. If you do, you might just get what you pay for. Your health is more valuable than your house or car, so do yourself a favor. Go ahead and invest in an experienced trainer/coach to make sure you're working with a credible and knowledgeable professional. It's easily one of the best decisions you'll ever make.

There are a few more things I want you to do. I want you to take out a calendar and schedule your gym time. Think about how many days a week you're prepared to dedicate to working out and make appointments with yourself. This will be your time. Lack of consistency is one of the reasons people never reach their goals. They're not consistent, in part, because they leave their workouts to chance. They go to the gym when they want to, or when they *feel* like it. This approach won't work if you want to be successful. Schedule your gym time just like you would a doctor's appointment, or a date with your significant other. Things are going to happen that are beyond your control and will potentially interfere with your training time. So, you might want to schedule an extra day.

You'll also want to think about the best time of the day to work out. If you're a morning person, consider hitting the gym before work, if your schedule allows it. If you'd rather go after you get off work, think about how the evening will flow in terms of family and household responsibilities. Do you have to cook dinner? Help the kids with homework? Spend time with your mate? These are just a few things to consider before you commit to evenings. Not to mention, most gyms are really crowded after work. So, if you don't like crowds, you may want to get up early.

Put your family members and friends on notice that you're embarking on a new journey, because you're going to need their support and understanding. Committing time to the gym, in some cases, means less time to spend with them. It's important that they understand why you're working out, and how it will impact their lives too. Hopefully, you'll get buy-in from them, so they can be active members of your support system.

If you haven't had a physical or a check-up recently, you'll need to call your doctor and schedule an appointment before you start training. Don't assume everything is alright just because you don't notice any symptoms. There are serious illnesses that people are unaware of until they visit the doctor's office. High blood pressure and diabetes are two of the most prevalent, and they can have a major impact on how you feel before, during, and after workouts. I've had clients who struggled to lose weight, and after getting checked out, discovered they had thyroid issues. Hormonal imbalances can make weight loss more challenging, but not impossible. Get a thorough exam to make sure there are no undiagnosed health issues.

One of my first clients, a retired teacher in her early 60's, decided it was time to act after coming from a doctor's appointment. Her doctor told her she needed to lose weight and she took him seriously. "Because of health concerns I need to be as active as possible. I already have hypertension and high cholesterol. I'm also a borderline diabetic with a family history of heart disease." We went through our initial training sessions, then the time came to talk about long-term or extended training. I did my presentation and after I told her what it would cost, I stopped to let her digest the information. I could see she was thinking about something. The wheels were turning. After a period of uncomfortable silence, she said, "OK, let's do it." I later asked her, "What were you thinking about?" She told me she was trying to figure out what she needed to move around, so she could make her monthly training payments. She decided to sacrifice some of her shopping, and a few other things, to make it work. She made the decision to put her health first and knew she couldn't do it alone.

She reached her weight loss goal and has drastically increased her strength and endurance. However, she readily admits that she still struggles with preparing meals ahead of time. "I'm not consistent with meal planning." She says. "Too many of my meals are put together at the last minute. I rely on the same foods, or I don't eat anything at all, which I know is not good." One of her early challenges, like many people, was working out alone and pushing herself. Over the years, she's made improvements and is much better at going to the gym on her own. She advises gym newbies to set small goals, and once you reach them, set new ones. "Start at your own pace and don't be distracted by what others are doing. You might not see changes right away but keep going!" We've worked together for several years now, and we continue to set and reach new goals.

CHAPTER 3

You Can't BE What You Don't EAT

Most of us know the difference between healthy food and junk food. This understanding alone, however, doesn't stop us from making unhealthy choices. Even if we make the decision to start eating better, we're often pulled back into our old habits. We fall victim to the overwhelming number of fast food restaurants, and our urges for sugar and salt. Temptation is everywhere, and willpower alone usually isn't enough to stop us. I did a little research, and you can do the same thing in your city. I decided to drive down a 3 mile stretch of one of the busiest avenues in my area. I wanted to see how many restaurants and convenience stores there were. *I counted 70!* That's an average of about 23 per mile. This partly explains why so many of us are overweight and obese. Keep in mind, most of them are fast food restaurants, and unfortunately, they're building more! If you're fighting food cravings and are trying to eat better, you don't stand a chance driving down roads like this one.

The food industry is interested in profits. They're going to do whatever is necessary to make money. Your health is *NOT* their top priority. What does that mean for you? It means you must advocate for your own health and well-being by educating yourself on what's in the food you eat, and how it affects your body. You're probably thinking "I've been eating this way for years and this is all I know!" I understand how you feel, but here's the question. Are your current eating habits moving you toward health and longevity, or toward sickness and pre-mature death? In other words, how are your habits working for you?

Just because you've been doing something for 20 or 30 years, it doesn't mean the behavior is good for you. Your parents and grand-parents cooked certain foods for you as a child, but some of those foods were very unhealthy. I know that's hard to hear, but it's the truth. In most cases, they did the best they could with the knowledge and resources they had. We now have a lot more information at our fingertips, so we're able to quickly research topics like carbs, protein, and fat. After you get the information, you still need to act on it. If you're like me, and you have a family history of diseases like diabetes and high blood pressure, it's time to take a hard look at what you're eating and change your attitude toward food.

Figuring out what to eat can be a tremendous challenge. Is red meat ok? What about gluten? What is gluten anyway? Should I limit my carbs? Add more protein? Fat is bad, right? Information overload causes many people to get frustrated, and once that happens it's easy to fall back into your old and familiar habits. That's why it's important to take things slowly and try not to make too many changes at once. Start by setting small goals. You'll need to practice the same patience and consistency you use in the gym, as you work to navigate the obstacles to healthy eating.

Developing better eating habits ultimately means challenging your current eating behavior and patterns. What's going on in your life that causes you to eat the way you do? Are you eating when you're not hungry? Do you eat to comfort yourself, when you feel stressed? Is there something about your schedule that sets you up to make bad choices?

Does someone else in your household do the grocery shopping? Do you use your children as an excuse to buy sweets and other junk food? In my experience, changing eating habits can be a real struggle. To make things worse, we lie to ourselves. We don't want to admit what's really going on. The truth is too painful, and we'd rather live in denial because the lie is comfortable and much easier to deal with. At least that's what we think.

Food sits at the center of our lives, and our obsession with it crosses racial and ethnic lines. When we get together to celebrate birthdays and holidays, we eat. When we go to sporting events or concerts, we eat. When we attend a marriage ceremony, we celebrate the union with food. When someone passes away, we mourn their loss with food. Everywhere you turn there's an opportunity to eat and load up more calories. Even if you're not hungry, your senses can be overwhelmed especially when you're out with friends and you're surrounded by food. It happens all the time.

The gas station is a perfect example of how obsessed we are with food. The truth is we don't really have gas stations anymore. We have food stops that just happen to sell gas too! I often go by one of these well-known gas stations for my morning coffee, and though they've started selling a little fresh fruit, that's not what I see most people buying. It's disheartening to watch people come in and get a 40-ounce soda for breakfast, along with a couple of doughnuts, chips, or cookies. As a matter of fact, the 40-ounce is probably conservative for some people.

The amount of sugar in these drinks is staggering. A 12-ounce soda alone has about 40 grams of sugar. Imagine taking a glass of water and mixing in about 10 teaspoons.

Would you drink it? Probably not, but that's basically what you're drinking every time you pop the top on that can of your favorite beverage. When you buy a 40 oz fountain drink, you're consuming close to 40 teaspoons of sugar. Let that sink in for a minute! I've met people over the years who drink a six-pack or more *every* day. If this is you, I recommend that you work on cutting back right away. The long-term impact on your health of consuming this much sugar is devastating.

What's even more heartbreaking is to see people walk in with their children and grab junk food first thing in the morning. As a former teacher, I'm very sensitive about children and good nutrition, because I know the impact it has on their performance in the classroom. A developing child can't be at her best without getting the proper vitamins and minerals she needs. We know the availability of junk food greatly contributes to the epidemic of childhood obesity and other illnesses, and the bad news is, things are getting worse!

If you're going to be successful at losing weight, you have to take eating just as seriously as your workouts. I recommend starting with 1 or 2 goals. For example, if you don't eat breakfast, work on eating a light meal every morning. If you're not drinking enough water, set a goal to increase your daily intake. If you eat out a lot, work on cooking more of your meals. Planning your meals ahead of time will get you thinking about what you eat and will save money.

Here's the question I want you to regularly ask yourself. *Was this week better than the last one?* If the answer is yes, then you're moving in the right direction. If the answer is no, then you've got to figure out where you went wrong and get back on track. You're not going to change years of bad eating overnight. It takes time, patience, and commitment to develop better habits. So, when you stumble and fall, *and you will*, don't be too hard on yourself. Get up, dust yourself off, and start again.

Keeping a food journal can be a very helpful tool because it provides accountability and gives you an ongoing record of what you're eating. If you're working with a trainer or coach, they'll need to know what your intake looks like before they can help you make adjustments. There are apps that allow you to record your daily intake, but I usually ask my clients to write their food down. There's something about the act of writing that makes it real. Many are shocked to find out how much they really eat, while others realize they're under-eating. Writing down what you eat also helps you discover patterns. Do you eat mostly during the day? Are you consuming most of your calories at night? Do your calories increase on the weekends? Knowing that you'll have to record it, brings a certain level of awareness to your food choices.

You may have heard the term *clean eating*. What does it mean to eat clean? If you ask 10 people, you'll probably get 10 different answers. Eating clean basically means avoiding or limiting foods that are heavily processed and packaged. I call it factory food because most of it is man-made. Focus on increasing the amount of *real* food you eat. I'm talking about fruits, vegetables, whole grains, etc. These foods give you energy and provide the body with valuable vitamins and minerals. I think it's important to make fruit and vegetables the foundation of your daily food intake, but you don't have to become a vegetarian to reap the benefits.

25

As you begin your journey toward healthier eating and reflect on your food journal, start by asking yourself a couple of questions. How much real food am I eating? How much of my intake is processed or packaged food? It doesn't matter where you are now. Examine your eating habits and begin to make the changes to start tilting the ratio of real to processed food in your favor. You can start doing this by adding a piece of fruit to breakfast or by eating a salad for lunch. Remember to take things one step at a time and set small goals. Trying to tackle too many things at once usually leads to frustration and failure.

Here's another thing to keep in mind. *No one eats clean all the time!* Everyone eats junk food. We all eat cookies, cake, chips, doughnuts, and pizza. Yes, even trainers and coaches! The difference is, fitness pros tend to eat healthy most of the time and work out more than the average person. So, the occasional piece of cake or slice of pizza, doesn't do as much damage. You don't have to deprive yourself of foods you like or eat clean all the time to get into shape, but you do have to make good decisions most of the time.

Please don't make the mistake of thinking you can work out, eat whatever you want, and still lose weight. I know many people who've tried this and while they're able to build strength and increase their endurance, they struggle to drop the extra pounds. Why? Because they have what's called a positive energy balance. That means despite all the hard work in the gym, they're still consuming more calories than they burn off. If you want to lose weight, you must create a negative energy balance by working off more calories than you eat and drink. There's no way around science. Don't be the person who wants to lose 30 pounds and three years later you're still working on it. If you want to successfully reach your goals, you don't have to be perfect, but you need to be serious about your food intake. Eat to live, eat to be healthy, eat to fuel your body, and eat to feel better! The weight will take care of itself.

Water intake is another component of good health that gets overlooked. Again, there's a lot of information out there about how much you should drink, so let's break it down. The amount of water you need each day is influenced by a few factors. One is exercise. Generally, the more intense the exercise is, the more water you'll need to drink. By the way, don't wait until you finish working out to start drinking. Start rehydrating *while* you work out! Another factor is the environment you live in. If you live in a warm climate, you're going to sweat more throughout the day, so you might need more water than someone living in a cooler location. Health conditions and medications can also affect how much water your body needs. Fortunately, fruit and vegetables also contain water, so make sure you consider them when examining your daily intake.

When I share this information people usually say, "Ok, I understand that, but how much do I need to drink?" As a general guideline, I usually recommend drinking about 2 liters a day along with your fruit and vegetables. I know people who drink more, but you should pay attention to your thirst and your needs. If two liters sounds like a lot, don't worry about it. Focus on improving your intake a little at a time. If you only drink one bottle, set a goal to drink two. If you're drinking two, go for three or four bottles. Don't let it overwhelm you, just work on doing better. Is it possible to drink too much water? Yes, but most people don't come anywhere near an amount that will jeopardize their health.

To set yourself up for nutritional success, I want you to spend some time in your kitchen. Believe it or not, many of us don't have the proper utensils and equipment to prepare healthy meals. Whether it's the right cutlery, a blender, a food processor, measuring cups, or storage containers, make sure your kitchen has the essentials. The next thing I want you to do is grab a big trash bag, open the refrigerator and cabinets, and start throwing out the junk food. Now you're probably saying to yourself, "I paid for that, I'm not throwing it out." "Can I just give it to someone else?" I wouldn't recommend giving it away to anyone else for the same reasons I don't want you to eat it. It's sugar, salt, and chemical filled junk, that does harm to your body and your health. Please throw it out, because it's too tempting to keep it in your house.

As you transition to healthier eating and exercise, sooner or later you're going to come across someone promoting the benefits of taking supplements. We're talking about a multi-billion-dollar industry that continues to expand each year. One of the reasons for this growth is people want faster results, and if we think a supplement will help us get there, we're more likely to try it. Fitness and health professionals continue to debate the effectiveness of supplements, and you certainly should do your own research before putting anything into your body. Please understand a supplement is supposed to be something you take in addition to your regular food intake. It's not supposed to take the place of eating good healthy food. Before you start taking a bunch of pills, capsules, and powders, the first step is to clean up your diet by consuming more fruit, vegetables, and whole foods. As you do that, you're likely to find you don't need to take anything else. There are some cases when your doctor may recommend taking a supplement to address a deficiency or other health issue. If you decide to take something on your own, always let your doctor know, especially if you're taking other medications.

One of my younger clients would be the first to admit that she's struggled with eating over the years. She's in her late 20's and works for a large aerospace company. As a child, she was involved in swimming, gymnastics, and soccer, but after 6th grade those activities slowed drastically. It really wasn't until her junior year in college that she started to become active again. Weight has been a constant struggle, and as a freshman in high school she almost reached 300 pounds. After graduating from college, she recommitted herself to getting in better shape and losing weight. She admits, "I haven't seen a number under 200 probably since middle school. It's been difficult to find clothes that fit and are in style." Like most of us, she struggles with portion control and food preparation, and she continues to work on changing her attitude about food. Her focus is changing her mindset, so that she's not eating for pleasure, but rather for sustenance.

She admits that she likes barbell work, but there are times when she's a little uncomfortable around what she calls "male buffies." These are the guys in the gym you hear making all kinds of noises and throwing weights around as they work out. She wishes someone would open an all-female gym with free weights, so women can focus on building their bodies without the distractions. When asked what advice she'd give to someone who is new to working out and wants to get in better shape, she recommends getting out of your comfort zone and trying new things. She also thinks being obsessed with the scale is a bad idea, and she cautions others to remember that results take time. "Don't compare yourself with anyone else and don't be intimidated, if it seems like everyone is doing better than you. I found a guy in my gym who is willing to work out with me from time to time, and I end up doing things I wouldn't do if I were there by myself."

I love her positive outlook and attitude. She has a quiet confidence that lets you know she's going to reach her goals. She doesn't let setbacks knock her out of the game, and she keeps fighting no matter what comes her way. Yes, her weight has been a challenge that she continues to deal with, but she's not letting it stop her from living and enjoying her life!

CHAPTER 4

To LIFT or Not to LIFT

The gym can be very intimidating if you don't have much experience lifting weights or using some of the newer cardio machines. When you walk in and see all the equipment, you think to yourself "Wow, I don't know where to start, or how to use any of this stuff." Don't panic. Most commercial gyms have trainers and other staff who will help you learn how to use the equipment, but don't expect to figure everything out on your first couple of trips. I've watched people over the years try to go it alone and end up getting hurt or developing bad form. If you want to get off to a good start, learn which movements are the most beneficial and will give you the best results. If you don't want to work with a trainer, you might be more comfortable talking to one of their clients. I would caution you to be careful about getting help from random members. Gyms are full of people with good intentions, but they don't necessarily know or practice correct form.

New members often wonder whether they should use machines or focus on free weights. This is a popular question and one that's worth discussing. Both can be beneficial as part of your overall program, but let's talk about machines first. These are the pieces of equipment you'll see in most gyms, that usually require you to sit and work a muscle in isolation. For example, a bicep curl machine focuses mostly on your biceps, but it doesn't work much else. Machines are a relatively safe way to start building strength and muscle endurance. They're also less intimidating than some of the free weight movements. Can you get results using machines? The short answer is yes. I know people who have reshaped their bodies using a few machines, doing cardio, and improving their eating habits.

Free weights are the way to really start sculpting your body because they give you more flexibility and variety. Some women are intimidated by lifting weights because they're worried about building too much muscle and looking masculine. Here's the good news. The typical woman is *never* going to look like a man. Women simply don't have the biological make-up for that to happen. Yes, you will run across women who are very muscular, and maybe that's not the look you want. The average woman, however, shouldn't worry. Lifting weights helps you build muscle, strengthen your bones and your joints, increase your endurance, and transform your body in ways you never imagined.

When it comes to free weights there are all kinds of movements and exercises you can do. I'm a big believer in doing movements that are going to give you the biggest bang for your buck. In other words, spend your time doing things that will build the most muscle and help burn the most calories. That's where compound movements come in. These are movements that allow you to work more than one muscle group at a time, because you bend more than one joint during the exercise. For example, when you squat you're bending at the hips, knees, and ankles. That means you're working your glutes (butt), quads (front thigh), hamstrings (back thigh), and calves. Your core and back are also involved. When you're at the bottom of a back squat, with some good weight on the bar, it's hard to find a muscle that's not contracting to help you stand up. There are times when you may want to work solely on your calves or triceps and there's nothing wrong with that. I just want you to understand the difference between isolation and compound movements.

So, if you're serious about losing body fat and building muscle, *it's a good idea to make squats, deadlifts, push-ups and pull-ups, part of your weekly regimen!* Why? The amount of muscle recruitment involved to perform these movements make them extremely effective at creating the body you want. As I mentioned, squats are basically a complete workout. Deadlifts work a lot of muscles too! They work your hamstrings, glutes, back, arms, core, and other muscles. Push-ups and pull-ups help build muscle and strength in your chest, back, shoulders, arms, and core.

For a beginner these movements might be a little intimidating. That's why it's important to get a good coach and learn how to do them correctly to avoid injury. I see people doing them wrong all the time, and as with most things in life, it's easier to learn how to do something right the first time.

Here's another thing to think about. As we move into our 30's, we start losing muscle mass. You can lose up to 5 pounds of muscle each decade, if you're not doing weight training. You may not notice the loss, because at the same time you're losing muscle, the scale is going up because you're gaining body fat. As we get older, we are completely unaware of what's happening to our muscle mass. Why do we need muscle? The obvious reason is to keep us strong and mobile, so we can move efficiently through our day. I had a client who mentioned that one of her co-workers had trouble getting up from a chair without holding on to something.

She's in her early 50's! She's been inactive for a long time, and as a result, has lost some of the strength she needs for basic activities. How many of us have elderly parents or relatives who struggle to make it through everyday tasks like getting out of bed, using the bathroom, or just walking? None of us want to be in that position. Starting a weight training program (no matter how old you are) will help strengthen your muscles, bones, and joints, and will help you stay vibrant and strong.

Let's talk a little about how weight training helps maximize fat loss. Muscle helps you maintain a more active and efficient metabolism, which helps you burn more calories. After a weight lifting session, your body will continue to burn calories *after* the workout is over. The length of this post-workout calorie burn depends on what kind of shape you're in and the intensity of the exercise. So, if weight loss is your goal, building muscle will help you get there! Don't be afraid to pack on as much as you can. Very few women, or men, walk around saying "I think I have too much muscle; this doesn't look right on me." Pick up some weights and go to work.

When you start a weight lifting program, expect to experience muscle soreness. How sore you get will depend, in part, on your level of fitness. If you've been inactive for a while, the soreness can be very uncomfortable in the beginning. After a few weeks of consistent training, you won't hurt nearly as much. Intermediate and advanced folks usually don't experience as much soreness unless they break their routine and do different exercises. What causes muscle soreness? Well, some soreness is unavoidable, but when you get so sore that it hurts to walk or get out of bed, it usually means you did too much. This is very common for beginners. When you have a goal and you're focused on it, the temptation is to work out as much as possible because we think more is better. Well, that's not always the case. Lifting weights too often can have a couple of negative side effects. First, the body doesn't get the time it needs to recover and rebuild properly. Weight training tears down your muscle fibers, and rest allows them to repair and grow back stronger. Skipping rest keeps your body under constant stress and will hinder your progress. Second, the lack of rest and recovery will impact your performance during future workouts. For example, if you work out hard really hard on Monday and decide to work the same muscles on Tuesday, you're likely to struggle. Why? Because your body hasn't had time to rest.

When it comes to cardiovascular exercise most gyms have an abundance of equipment including treadmills, elliptical machines, stair climbers, rowing machines, and bikes. You can get a good workout, and burn body fat too, if you have the right approach. If you like using the elliptical, go for it. But, don't do it the same way every time. The first time go ahead and work at a moderate pace for 15 to 20 minutes. The next time switch things up a little. Instead of working at the same pace, alternate the resistance and/or incline. You can do the first couple of minutes at a moderate level, and then increase the resistance to a level that gets your heart rate up. Basically, you're raising your heart rate and then slowing it down. You'll do this for the entire time you're on the elliptical. You can do this kind of interval training on any piece of equipment, or you can do the same thing if you're outside at a park or a track. Walk for a few minutes, switch to a jog or run, and then go back to walking.

You can put cardio into two categories. LISST (Low Intensity Steady State Training) and IIIT (High Intensity Interval Training). Both forms of cardio have benefits and you can make both part of your program. The steady pace method is low impact, easier on the joints, and helps build endurance. The interval method helps burn more body fat, but it will also challenge you mentally. It's this challenge that forces the body and *mind* to get stronger because working out is as much mental, as it is physical. We tend to stop when we get that uncomfortable tightness or fatigue in our muscles, or if it gets a little harder to breathe. It's human nature to stop when we get outside our comfort zone. Don't get me wrong, there are times when you need to stop to rest, but there are also times when you need to push through! Staying comfortable won't get you the results you're looking for. If you want to change your body, you'll have to do some things you don't like. The stronger you get mentally, the better chance you'll have to succeed.

I get questions all the time about taking classes like Yoga, Pilates, Cycling, and Zumba. I think you should take them if you want to. If you do things you enjoy, you're more likely to stick with a workout program long term. Yoga and Pilates are great for developing core strength and increasing flexibility, which will help with weight training. Cycling and Zumba are good for building cardio-vascular endurance and improving coordination. By taking classes, you'll also build a sense of community with other people who are working toward some of the same goals. One of the problems I do see with classes is some people rely on them exclusively. So, as you develop your program, with the help of a trainer or coach, include activities you enjoy along with regular weight training.

One of my success stories, a 49-year-old support analyst for a major banking firm, became a big believer in the power of weight training. She explains, "When I started, I just took cycling classes and I walked on the treadmill. Now I work with a trainer and do a little cardio on my off days." She does squats, deadlifts, bench press, pull ups, etc., and in a relatively brief period she reached her initial goal of losing 20 pounds. We also drastically improved her strength and increased her muscle mass. Like many women, she's motivated by wanting to look good in her clothes (especially her bathing suits). As she fast approaches the big 50, maintaining good health is also important to her.

She is an example of how you don't have to be perfect to reach your goals and change your body. You just need to be committed! She admits, "My challenge is carbs like pasta and warm rolls. I try to avoid them as much as possible, but there are times when I fall off the wagon and sometimes I fall hard." Carbs are an issue for most us, but she recognizes her struggle and works to limit the damage. We train a couple of days a week at 6:00 a.m. So, while most people are still asleep, she's putting in work. When you're committed you'll do whatever it takes to reach your goals. Her advice to beginners is "Don't give up! It gets hard and sometimes you'll want to quit, but you have to keep going. Dig deep and push yourself. Look in the mirror and tell yourself that you're in control of your destiny, and you want weight loss to be a part of that. It's a lifestyle change, but it's so worth it."

Though she's a bit of a perfectionist, I appreciate her desire to do things right, especially when it comes to form. She had a shoulder injury that she's still recovering from, but it didn't stop us from working on other things while it healed. If you work out long enough, eventually you're going to strain, sprain, or injure something. That's part of training. Warming up, stretching, and rest, will decrease the odds, but it will happen. Deal with it and keep going.

CHAPTER 5

It's All **WORTH** *the* **WEIGHT**

As a country, we are in big trouble! Obesity rates in the United States have reached epidemic proportions. Researchers tell us that over one-third of adults in the U.S. are obese. When you add in those who are classified as overweight, more than 50% of the population is dealing with some type of weight problem. The number of obese children has *tripled* since the 1970's, reaching over 12 million. Let that sink in for a moment. As a society, we are getting bigger and bigger, and our children are dealing with health issues once reserved for adulthood. Type 2 diabetes among children used to be a rare occurrence, but each year thousands of kids are diagnosed with this deadly disease. When extra fat surrounds our organs, the odds of developing heart disease, high cholesterol, or cancer, increase dramatically. The physical impact of obesity can be devastating but carrying too much weight can also have a tremendous impact on your self-esteem and confidence.

We have a way, particularly in the United States, of making people feel lesser because they're overweight. Carrying around extra pounds can be uncomfortable, and some may find it unattractive, but your value as a human being isn't diminished because of what the scale says. Despite the weight, you still have gifts and talents to share with the world and improving your health will put you in a better position to fulfill your purpose. Looking good in your clothes won't hurt either!

Weight loss can be overwhelming, especially when you don't know where to start. The overabundance of diets and weight loss programs only add more confusion to an already challenging task. Most diets will work in the short term, because whether it's low carb, low fat, or high protein, the one thing diets have in common is that they restrict your caloric intake. So, you always lose weight in the short term, because you're eating fewer calories. The problem is you're not going to stay on a diet forever, and as soon as you resume eating other foods your calories go up and the weight comes back. The challenge is to find a way to eat that's consistent with your goals, and a way you can maintain for the rest of your life.

Many people ask, "Don't I need to count calories to lose weight?" Calorie counting can be very inaccurate, but it can provide you with some information about how much you eat. It also makes you pay more attention to your choices and gets you reading food labels. Some of my clients use apps because of the convenience, and it helps hold them accountable for their food intake. But, I don't stress them out about counting calories. My goal is to get them focused on eating nutrient dense foods instead of the high calorie, low nutrient alternatives. What am I talking about? Vegetables are a great example of foods that are low in calories, but very high in the vitamins and minerals your body needs to function properly. On the other hand, chocolate cake or ice cream may taste good, but these foods are very high in calories and very low in vitamins and minerals. Limiting, or getting rid of junk food is crucial if you want to lose weight and maintain it.

Probably one of the most overlooked ways of controlling your food intake is portion control. We're so accustomed to just sitting down and eating, that we don't pay much attention to how *much* we eat. We're conditioned to finish what's on our plates even if we're not hungry. Practicing portion control will obviously limit the amount of food you eat, and it will help you pay attention to your hunger cues. You'll start to realize that you can eat less and still feel satisfied. One of the easiest ways to start is to eat from a smaller plate or dish. It takes getting used to, but it works. The portion sizes at restaurants can be huge. When you eat out, you can ask for a carry-out box when you order your food. Once your meal arrives, go ahead and box up half of it and save it for the next day. When you cook at home, you can use a scale or measuring cups to portion out your food. The point is to find a way to exercise control over how much food you eat so you can lose weight.

In addition to portion control, I highly recommend slowing down when you eat. Put the fork down between bites and enjoy your food. Most of us eat too fast because we're usually in a hurry, but it takes around 20 minutes for your brain to let your stomach know you've had enough. If you cram everything down in 10 minutes, this natural process doesn't have time to work. You also want your food to properly digest which means it's important to chew it completely before you swallow.

If you're struggling to shed pounds, it's important to understand that you're on a journey, and it takes time and patience to reach your destination. It's not realistic to expect to lose 50 pounds in a month. I've worked with clients who have lost 10-15 pounds in their first month, but that doesn't happen very often. It's realistic to expect to lose 1-2 pounds a week. It may not sound like much but think about it this way.

Losing a consistent 1-2 pounds a week results in 4-6 pounds in a month. Over a 6-month period that means dropping between 24 and 36 pounds. I think most people would take that. Along with losing the weight, you'll lose inches and your clothes are going to fit better. As a matter of fact, you're going to need new ones.

Here's something else to consider. Remember line graphs in math class? It's been a while for most of us! To refresh your memory, they basically show how something increases or decreases over time. For example, you can use a graph to chart strength improvements, or you can track your weight over the course of a year. Let's say it's January and you want to lose 60 pounds by December. Each month you plot your weight on the graph and connect the dots from previous months. Even if you reach your goal by December, you probably won't have a straight line showing the same amount of weight loss every month. You may have months when you lose 8 pounds or more, but there may also be months when you only lose 3 to 4. You might even gain a pound or two. Ultimately, it's about where you finish, not the fluctuations you experience month to month. Just like a pilot makes course corrections during a flight, you'll have to do the same during your journey.

Many people have asked, "Do I need to weigh myself daily?" The answer is no. I don't have a problem with scales because they provide accountability and let you know if you're moving in the right direction. However, your weight can change every day, and I don't want you getting frustrated if your number temporarily goes up. Things can especially be volatile in the first couple of months. This is the time when you'll struggle the most with your eating and getting used to a new workout routine. I recommend stepping on the scale once a week, because this is often enough to let you know how things are going without driving yourself crazy. At the end of the day, the scale is just one indicator. The scale can't measure improvements in your strength and endurance. It can't tell you how much better your clothes fit. It can't measure your confidence, your commitment, or your will. So, don't obsess about your weight. If you make better food choices and work out regularly, the weight will take care of itself.

Every now and then someone will ask, "What can I do to get rid of this back fat? Too much fat on the arms, legs, and back is annoying, but as I mentioned earlier, extra fat around the mid-section is a major health concern. This is where your kidneys, intestines, pancreas, liver, and other organs are located. Extra fat in these areas can increase the chances of developing diabetes, high blood pressure, and heart disease. While genetics may play a role in determining where you accumulate fat, your genes don't necessarily have the final say. No matter what DNA was passed on to you, you can still reach your goals by working hard and committing to healthier eating.

If you want to get rid of that annoying back or arm fat, the key is to work everything. Work your entire body. Don't just focus on one or two body parts. Decreasing your overall body fat percentage means that you'll drop fat from your mid-section, your back, your arms, and your legs. Now that doesn't mean you need to do a full body workout every time you step into the gym. If you're only working out 2 or 3 days a week, go for it. You'll have enough time to rest and recover. On the other hand, if you train more frequently, doing a full body workout might not be the best way to go.

Don't fall victim to taking shortcuts to drop body fat. Working out in a plastic suit or wrapping yourself in plastic wrap, are not effective ways to lose weight, no matter how many people you see doing it. I witnessed a young man nearly pass out one day in the locker room at my gym. He wore a plastic suit *under* his sweat pants and hoodie while he worked out, and then he went into the sauna for another 30 minutes. He clearly was in distress, as he sat on the bench sweating profusely and looking disoriented. Luckily, there happened to be a nurse in the gym, and she was able to look after him. Things turned out fine, but it could have been a very dangerous situation.

The lack of patience, in part, is what drives people to look for ways to speed up the process. It's not about how fast you can lose weight. The key is doing it in a way that you can maintain over the long term. I know people who decided to have weight loss surgery, and while this may seem like an extreme step, I understand how people get to the point where they feel this is their best option. I'm not going to pass judgement, but it's important to do your own research to make sure you have a thorough understanding of the procedure and the risks involved. If you're expecting surgery to be a magical solution to your weight problem, you're going to be disappointed. The weight *will* come back, if you don't make the necessary lifestyle changes to keep it off. Research suggests that most people who lose a lot of weight quickly, will gain it back. That means that surgery is often just another short-term and expensive fix.

I train an analyst for a fleet management company, who has struggled with her weight, but hasn't fallen prey to quick-fix solutions. She admittedly sits for hours while at work and says her company's celebrations, "are usually centered around food." This can be a huge challenge, because workplace celebrations typically include sugar-filled foods with lots of calories. In addition, co-workers pressure her by saying things like "a little bit won't hurt you," or "you're going to the gym anyway so enjoy it." If you haven't developed the discipline to say no, these celebrations can really sidetrack you and hinder your progress.

She's spent the last 20 years riding the weight loss rollercoaster. She acknowledges that, "After high school I became very inactive and didn't do much in the way of working out for years. When I attempted to get things going regularly, I would fall off the wagon and stay off for years at a time." In 2009 she started working out with a well-known fitness company for women. She was hooked and believed she had finally found something she enjoyed. "It was the ideal place for me to begin because the environment was non-threatening and encouraging." In 2010, she was introduced to Zumba and immediately became hooked! She took as many classes as she could, and in 2011 she became a certified Zumba Fitness instructor. "The decision to become an instructor was for me, but also to encourage those who look like me. I know from personal experience that walking into a class where all of the people are fit can be discouraging, so I wanted to be somewhat of a role model for those working to lose weight."

She remains focused on her goal of losing 100 pounds, and she works to include weight training along with cardio work. She struggles with following a consistent eating and workout plan, as many people do, but she remains optimistic and keeps going. I asked what advice she would give someone just starting out and her reply was, "You have to stick with it. Most any program will work, if you work it. The results will come, but we are far too impatient and give up before we see change." She's right! We want to see results right away and don't stick with it long enough to get them. The road to fitness is a long journey, and you're going to have to pay some dues to reach your goals. Fitness sure ain't free.

CHAPTER 6

The MUSCLE that MATTERS Most

A holistic approach is necessary if you want to have lasting health. That means addressing the mental components of health, as well as the physical. The physical challenges you'll face will demand mental toughness and resilience. Working out consistently for months and years isn't easy, and your commitment will be tested in ways you can't imagine. A fitness journey is like climbing a mountain. I've never done it before, but I'm sure those who have, will tell you it's just as tough and demanding as it looks. Imagine standing at the bottom of a huge mountain and looking up toward the peak knowing that's your destination. It must be an amazing and overwhelming site.

Successful climbers all have one thing in common. *No matter what happened they kept climbing.* Did they run into obstacles? Yes. Did they have to take alternate routes to get to the top? Yes. Did they need the support of other climbers? Yes. Of course! So, here's the lesson. Don't worry about things that get in your way. Don't worry about setbacks. Don't worry about people who try to sabotage your efforts, and don't worry about failing. Stand at the bottom of your mountain, look up, and no matter what comes your way, stay focused on your goals and keep climbing until you reach the TOP!

Where is the top, and how will you know when you reach it? Your top is different from everyone else's, because the top represents *your* physical, mental, and spiritual best. It

47

means living a healthy lifestyle and liberating yourself from toxic food, toxic people, and other negative influences. It means living a life of purpose and integrity. Living in a way that respects your health and the environment. Here are some questions to consider. What does my top look like? How close am I to reaching it? Am I doing what's necessary to get there? What do I need to do differently?

Building your mental muscles requires you to set aside time just as you would for working out. I highly recommend meditation as a tool to help you do this. It will increase your focus and help you develop more discipline. If you've never meditated before, don't get frustrated if you struggle with it in the beginning. Most people do. There are all kinds of resources out there to help you. There are books, DVD's, phone apps, and more. Just like your exercise program, it only works if you work it.

The goal of meditation is to quiet your mind, but don't confuse it with prayer. Think of prayer as communication from you to the universe (God). Meditation, on the other hand, is the universe communicating with you. The challenge is to be still, so you can receive the messages meant for you. With our daily responsibilities and activities, it's easy to miss out on valuable information, unless we take some time to *tune in*.

Before you start meditating, there are a couple of things you should do. First, figure out what time works best for you. Is it in the morning before work, or on your lunch break? Maybe the best time is after work? Next, think about the setting. Choose a place that's quiet and gives you the best chance to avoid interruptions. Some people like meditating at home, while others prefer being outdoors. You might like complete silence, or you may want to listen to soothing sounds like ocean waves or rainfall. Keep in mind, there's no right or wrong body position for meditation, so I suggest you discover what's comfortable for you. It might be sitting on the floor with your legs crossed or relaxing in your favorite chair. The goal is to find what works and go with it.

What's this "quiet your mind" thing about? It means emptying your mind of all thoughts and concerns. During the day, our minds are constantly racing and jumping from one thing to the next. What do I have to do at work? What time do I pick up the kids? What's for lunch? What's for dinner? What errands do I have to run? What am I doing after work? What time am I going to the gym? Our minds are constantly processing information, and there are very few opportunities throughout the day to stop and be still. Meditation is your opportunity to zone out and give your brain a break. Just as your other muscles get stronger after they recover from a tough workout, your brain will do the same thing. You'll emerge from meditation refreshed and focused.

Sitting still for 15 or 20 minutes, and not thinking about anything, is hard for most people. It may take a while to get to a point where you feel like you're doing it well. You might have to start with 5 minutes and work from there. In the beginning, the thoughts will come fast and furious, but when you catch yourself thinking, just stop and go back to it.

I've tried all kinds of things to quiet my mind. What seems to work best for me is to focus on my breathing. I inhale deeply, hold it for a few seconds, and then exhale. Sometimes I play meditation music to help me relax and create the right atmosphere. No matter where you meditate, there will be interruptions from time to time, especially if you do it outside. Again, don't get frustrated if a plane flies overhead or if you notice a car speed by. Don't give up just because you hear noise from the next room, or the dog is barking. Focus on your breathing and keep going.

Once you begin meditating on a regular basis, you'll start to notice a few things. I discovered that meditating before work has a very positive impact on my day. I'm more patient and less likely to become irritated by things that happen. It puts me in a better mood, and I feel more optimistic about life in general. It also helps me stay focused on my goals and the daily actions I need to take to reach them. People who meditate regularly experience all kinds of mental and *physical* benefits. Research has shown, among other things, that regular meditation lowers blood pressure, increases your energy level, and strengthens your immune system.

The ability to lock in and focus is important because change is not easy. There will be days that you don't feel like working out. Some days you'll get to the gym and realize you're not motivated to do anything. They'll be days when you'd rather go out to eat with friends. Mental toughness and discipline allow you to push through and get things done, even when you're not in the mood. I've worked with several clients over the years who displayed amazing amounts of mental strength. It showed in the way they dealt with adversity, the way they pushed through workouts, and how they fought back from injury.

Learning how to challenge yourself during workouts really pays off. Most people tend to stop when they start to get tired. This is exactly when you need to push yourself to do a little more. For example, there are a couple of people at my gym who do a plank routine a few times a week. A plank is a core building exercise that you do lying on your stomach and supporting your weight on your elbows and feet. They hold each plank for 90 seconds and then rest before the next one. They usually do about 3 rounds. After watching them do this for months, I decided to ask them, "When are you going to increase the time or make it tougher?" I asked because it was clear that they could do more if they wanted to, but like many people, they got comfortable with their routine and stopped giving themselves that extra push.

Your progress will stall on any exercise, if you don't continue to give your body more resistance. So, if you're doing planks and can hold them for a minute, go ahead and push for another 10 or 15 seconds. If you're struggling to do 1 minute, the extra time might seem like an eternity, but you can do it! If you take this approach, you'll develop a stronger mind and a stronger body. Sometimes we need to remind ourselves that workouts are about working, not playing around. By the time you leave the gym, you should be tired. You don't have to feel exhausted, but you should feel like you've done something.

Because the mind usually wants to give up before the body does, re-programing or rewiring your brain is key. Try this. When you pull into the parking lot of your gym, park the car, turn off the engine, and sit there before you go in. Spend a few minutes feeding your mind positive and affirming messages. Visualize yourself going through your workout and crushing it. See yourself running a few extra minutes on the treadmill. Picture yourself doing a couple of extra pull-ups or push-ups. Believe you can do more than your mind tells you. I tell my clients all the time, "You're tougher and stronger than you think you are." I believe that and so should you!

Another approach is to start doing things that scare you. In other words, face your fears. If you're afraid of heights, face it by going in a tall building, or any place that allows you to confront the anxiety you feel from high places. If you're afraid of water, face the fear by learning how to swim. If you're claustrophobic, face it by putting yourself in a tight space like a crowded train or bus. Don't misunderstand what I'm saying. There are some legitimate reasons why we fear certain things, and I don't want to suggest that overcoming them is easy. You should absolutely spend some time thinking about where the fear comes from and how it developed. After you've done that, go ahead and tackle it head on. Think about how you're going to feel once you overcome your fear. Think about how accomplished and empowered you'll feel.

Hopefully, these feelings will carry over into the gym, and you'll start pushing yourself further than you think you can go. Success in the gym spills over into other parts of your life too. People who are healthy and fit are often more confident in the workplace and in their personal lives. They walk and talk a certain way. They respond to adversity differently than most. They're climbers and they don't waste time *thinking* about how tall the mountain is, they get to it!

CHAPTER 7

Are You IN or OUT

When I sit down with potential clients for the first time, I ask questions about their fitness history, eating habits, health issues, goals, etc. One of the most important things I ask them to do is gauge their commitment level on a scale of 1 to 10. Anything under an 8 tells me their commitment is a little soft, and they may be struggling to find their motivation. On the other hand, an 8 or higher lets me know they're focused and clear about what they want. Of course, *saying* you're committed, doesn't make it so. It's easy to sit down with a health professional and say what you think they want to hear. Ultimately, your commitment is measured by what you do day in and day out.

Even with a high commitment level, obstacles will pop up from time to time. You must be willing to go over them, around them, or through them, to reach your goals. Here's something I really want you to hear. *You don't have to be a 10 to win!* Even if you're a 5 or 6, go ahead and get started. After you begin to see results and feel better about yourself, your commitment level will rise. I want you to think about where you are today. What's your number? How committed are you to changing your lifestyle? How committed are you to working out 3 to 4 days a week? How committed are you to changing your eating habits? Are you willing to sacrifice time with friends and family? Lifestyle change is serious business, and without commitment you'll be like a plastic bag blowing in the wind. You'll be out of control and all over the place.

Managing the space between your ears, or what I call your *inner game,* is crucial and will help strengthen your commitment. I'm talking about the things we tell ourselves and the thoughts floating around in our heads. Is your mind full of positive thoughts, or is it filled with negative chatter? Do you spend time visualizing the body and life you want to create? If you're not doing this, it's important to start now.

If you want to lose 50 pounds, start by first *seeing* yourself weighing less than you do now. Visualize how you'll look in that new pair of jeans or that outfit you like. Think about how other people are going to react once they see the new you. Think about the things you'll be able to do once you lose the weight. Regular visualization allows you to create what you want mentally before it happens physically. I suggest you practice visualization as often as possible, because feeding your subconscious mind with positive and self-affirming thoughts, is a powerful way to combat the negative energy you get from others and the negative thoughts you feed yourself.

You might be asking yourself, "What does this have to do with me losing weight or improving my health?" The answer is *everything.* Whether you realize it or not, your current reality is a result of the thoughts that have saturated your subconscious over the last few years or even decades. So, whatever is going on in your life now, you created or attracted it. What we think about most is what shows up in our lives. How does this relate to health? We spend too much time thinking about what we don't want, instead of focusing our minds on the new body we want to create. The goal is to start reprogramming your mind with positive thoughts and images, so it can start working for you.

As you work to rewire your brain, be careful about how you process and interpret information. Even if you do your best to guard against negative thoughts, you can't keep everything out. You can't stop a well-meaning family member or friend from saying something hurtful. You can't control what others say, but you can control how you respond to it. For example, someone might respond negatively when they hear about your weight loss goal. Maybe they respond that way because they've heard you talk about losing weight before and you failed. Here's the thing. It doesn't matter what *they* think, it's about what *you* think. You can choose to allow their comments to tear you down, or you can use their words to motivate and fuel you to push harder. This journey is not only about strengthening your body, it's also about training and strengthening your mind!

This leads to another crucial point. No matter how well things are going and how much progress you make, at some point during your journey, life will happen. You might get sick or injured. You may have a death in your family. You might lose your job, or your hours might change. There are several potential setbacks that may come your way, and some of them may consume much of your free time. When adversity strikes, working out may become less of a priority.

Keep in mind that exercise is a great stress reliever, and when things become chaotic, this is the time when you'll need those workouts the most. It will help take your mind off things for a while and help recharge your batteries. The challenge you'll face is finding the time, but if you're creative and committed you'll figure out how to make it work. You can get a good workout in 15 to 20 minutes, if you know what to do. If your job has a gym, that may be an option for you. You might even have to dust off that equipment in your basement. Do whatever it takes to make it happen, because life is not going to stop.

Be very mindful about how you eat during periods of decreased activity. If you're not able to work out, you won't burn off as many calories throughout the day. I know people who gained weight after long breaks from the gym and, in some cases, the gain was a result of failing to monitor their eating habits. A few weeks of bad eating, along with the stress of dealing with difficult circumstances, can wreak havoc on your waistline.

Whatever situation you find yourself in, remember it's temporary, and you will get back on track. The goal is to manage things the best you can until things return to normal. One client, who works as a high school science teacher, initially lost about 30 pounds after we started working together. We were right at that magical 200-pound mark and getting ready to break through. By the way, getting under 200 pounds is a big deal for people who haven't been there in years! She got injured on the job and worked through rehab, but since then she's struggled to get back on track. She lost a lot of her motivation and was feeling down for a while, but her resilience got her back on track again. She was sailing along and out of nowhere, life happened. So, start preparing yourself now, so you'll be able to navigate the roadblocks that come your way.

Another client endured countless surgeries and medical conditions over the years. I've never seen anything like it. She is one of the toughest people I've ever met. I really don't know how she does it. There are many days when she doesn't want to work out, but *she feels like she has to.* It makes her feel better, keeps her body relatively strong, and keeps her mind off the medical issues she deals with daily.

I frequently run into people who, for one reason or another, haven't worked out in a while. I usually ask them how they've been, and they typically respond by explaining what's going on in their lives and why they've been away. There are times when I jump in and say, "I understand" or "I get it." I want them to know, they don't have to explain why they missed time. What's important is, they found their way back to the gym and hit the reset button. That is why long-term thinking is so important. Where are you going to be in 5 years? 10 years? What do you want to look like? What do you want to be able to do? How do you want to feel? If you take the long view and understand that health and fitness is a process, you'll expect to hit the reset button, and you won't get as frustrated. Instead, you'll re-focus on your goals and keep going.

I made the decision to commit my life to help people build new bodies and reclaim their lives. Most of my days start very early. I get up, clean up, eat breakfast, and make my way to work. I usually arrive to a gym that's bustling with people in the middle of their morning workouts. Some of them lift weights, some run on treadmills, some ride bikes, and others take classes. It's inspiring to see so many people, up so early, working to get into shape. These people are *doing* it! They regularly show up and put in the work. As you start or reset your fitness journey, don't worry about getting everything right in the beginning. It's hard to pull it all together at once. *You can mess up, but don't give up!* Some weeks you'll complete your workouts but fall off with meal planning. There will be weeks when your meal preparation is on point, but you miss a couple of workouts. Don't sweat it, just keep going and do better.

Working as a trainer and coach have been extremely rewarding, and I've learned valuable lessons from the countless people I've worked with. Helping a client lose weight, get stronger, lower their blood pressure, or just increase their energy level, is a humbling experience. Each time I sit down with someone new, I'm awed by the privilege of helping them make lifestyle changes that will hopefully have a major impact on their health. I hope that you found something of value in this book that you can grab hold of and use immediately. There are people waiting to support you once you make the decision to climb your mountain. Don't forget to enjoy the journey and I can't wait to *See YOU at the TOP!*

ABOUT THE AUTHOR

Coach Obasi is a Certified Personal Trainer, Nutrition Coach, and Fitness Nutrition Specialist. He's spent the last 7 years working with clients primarily in St. Louis Missouri. Before beginning his career as a fitness professional, he spent 12 years working as an educator mostly at the elementary school level. Coach Obasi is dedicated to helping people develop healthier lifestyles and as a borderline diabetic, is particularly passionate about helping people lose weight and get their blood sugar under control.

If you're interested in health coaching or you want to book Coach Obasi for a speaking engagement, you can reach him at coachobasi@gmail.com or visit www.coachobasi.com

Made in the
USA
Columbia, SC